Accept Our Differences

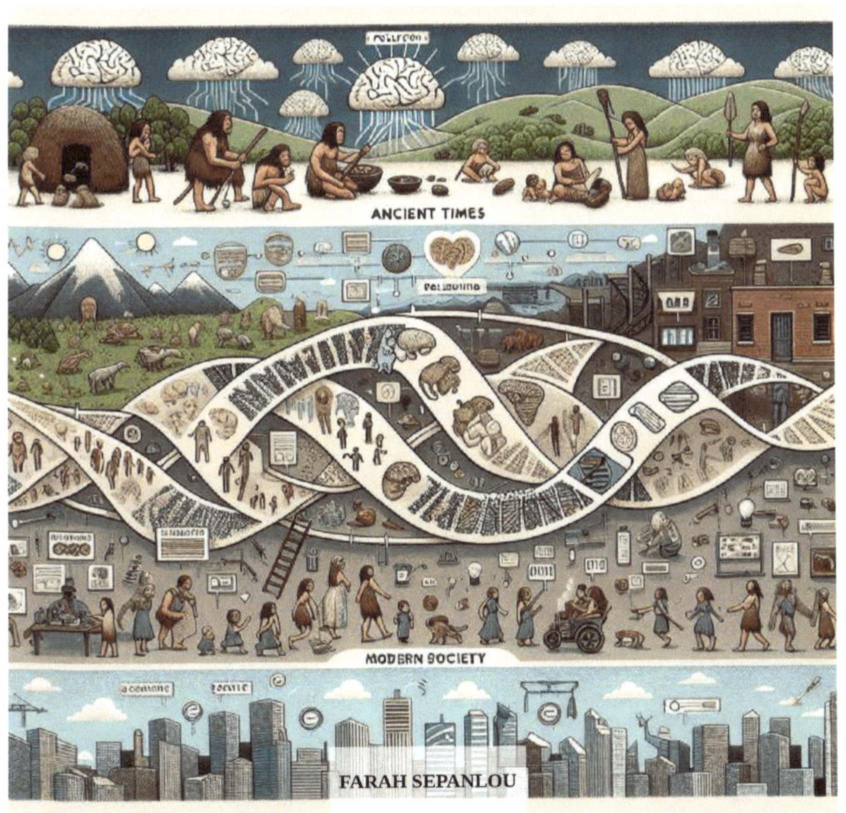

SUMMARY

1

The Foundations of Gender Differences

1.1 Understanding Intellectual Differences Between Genders

The exploration of intellectual differences between genders is not just a matter of academic curiosity but a crucial step towards understanding the complex interplay of biology, environment, and societal expectations that shape cognitive abilities and preferences. This nuanced understanding contributes significantly to the broader context of gender studies by highlighting how these differences influence personal relationships, professional choices, and societal roles.

Research indicates that on average, women tend to excel in verbal tasks and possess strong non-linear thinking capabilities. This proficiency can be seen in activities that require quick thinking and the ability to connect disparate ideas, such as in creative arts or language-based subjects. Conversely, men often show a predilection for math-based activities and exhibit strengths in linear thinking processes. This is evident in fields requiring step-by-step problem solving, such as engineering or computer science.

Emotional intelligence plays a vital role in interpersonal interactions and decision-making processes. Studies suggest that women generally display higher levels of emotional skills, which include empathy, emotional recognition, and emotional regulation. These skills are invaluable in professions and roles that demand high levels of interpersonal communication and care. On the other hand, men are frequently found to have superior spatial reasoning skills. This ability enhances performance in tasks involving navigation, three-dimensional manipulation, and abstract spatial analysis—skills particularly useful in architecture, surgery, and certain branches of physical sciences.

The distinction extends to motor skills as well; where men typically demonstrate stronger gross motor skills beneficial in sports or tasks requiring physical strength. Women excel in fine motor skills which are critical for tasks demanding precision and detail-oriented work such as writing, needlework, or surgery.

These intellectual differences between genders have evolutionary roots tied to the division of labor among early human societies where survival hinged on complementary skill sets between males and females. However, it's imperative to recognize that these are general trends rather than strict binaries; individuals may possess abilities typically associated with the opposite gender.

In contemporary society, the traditional roles based on these intellectual predispositions are increasingly blurred. The focus has shifted towards leveraging individual strengths regardless of gender. This evolution reflects a deeper understanding that intellectual capabilities are diverse and multifaceted within each gender group.

- Verbal vs Mathematical Abilities: Highlighting how each gender generally excels in different types of cognitive tasks.

- Emotional Intelligence vs Spatial Reasoning: Exploring the implications of these differing strengths on career choices and personal development.

- Fine vs Gross Motor Skills: Understanding how these physical abilities impact daily activities and professional competencies.

This comprehensive examination underscores the importance of recognizing intellectual differences not as limitations but as opportunities for synergy within diverse teams and relationships. By valuing these varied perspectives and abilities, society can foster more inclusive environments where every individual has the chance to thrive based on their unique strengths.

1.2 Evolutionary Perspectives on Gender Roles

The evolutionary perspective on gender roles offers a compelling framework for understanding the historical underpinnings of gender differences and how they have shaped societal norms and individual behaviors over millennia. This approach posits that many of the psychological and behavioral differences observed between men and women can be traced back to the distinct roles they played in early human societies, which were primarily driven by the necessities of survival and reproduction.

From an evolutionary standpoint, men often assumed roles that required physical strength, spatial awareness, and risk-taking behaviors. These roles included hunting, territory defense, and tool-making. Such activities not only demanded considerable physical prowess but also fostered skills like strategic planning and competitive behavior—traits that are often more pronounced in modern males. This alignment of ancient survival strategies with contemporary male tendencies highlights the deep-rooted nature of some gender-specific attributes.

Conversely, women's roles centered around childbearing, nurturing, and community bonding activities such as gathering plant-based foods, preparing meals, and caring for children. These responsibilities cultivated skills in social communication, empathy, multitasking, and cooperation—qualities that tend to be more developed in females even today. The emphasis on communal living and shared childcare among early humans further reinforced these traits, underscoring the evolutionary basis for women's strong interpersonal abilities.

This evolutionary lens also sheds light on mate selection processes where traits deemed beneficial for survival were favored. For instance, males displaying bravery or resourcefulness would have been attractive to females seeking protection and provision for their offspring. Similarly, females adept at social bonding and nurturing would appeal to males looking for partners who could ensure the well-being of their children.

- Physical Strength vs Nurturing: Illustrating how traditional roles influenced the development of gender-specific strengths.

- Spatial Awareness vs Social Communication: Comparing cognitive abilities shaped by ancient survival strategies.

- Risk-Taking vs Cooperation: Contrasting behavioral tendencies rooted in prehistoric division of labor.

In conclusion, while modern society has evolved beyond the strict confines of these ancient roles—thanks to technological advancements and changing social norms—the legacy of our evolutionary past continues to influence gender dynamics today. Recognizing this influence is crucial not only for understanding inherent gender differences but also for addressing contemporary issues related to gender equality and inclusivity. By examining these deep-seated origins, we gain insights into how best to leverage diverse strengths within both genders for mutual benefit in personal relationships, professional environments, and broader societal contexts.

1.3 The Impact of Society and Culture on Gender Expectations

The intricate web of society and culture plays a pivotal role in shaping gender expectations, influencing everything from individual behavior to institutional norms. This complex interplay not only perpetuates traditional gender roles but also challenges and reshapes them in the face of evolving societal values. Understanding the impact of society and culture on gender expectations requires a deep dive into various facets, including historical context, media representation, educational systems, and legislative frameworks.

Historically, societal structures have been built around distinct gender roles, with men typically occupying positions of power and women relegated to subordinate roles. These historical precedents have laid the groundwork for contemporary gender expectations, embedding stereotypes into the fabric of daily life. However, as societies evolve, there is a noticeable shift towards more fluid and inclusive understandings of gender. This evolution reflects changing cultural narratives that challenge traditional binaries and advocate for greater equality.

Media representation is another critical area where the impact of society and culture on gender expectations is evident. Television shows, movies, advertisements, and social media platforms often reinforce or challenge societal norms related to gender. For instance, the portrayal of women in empowered roles can challenge traditional stereotypes and inspire change. Conversely, perpetuating clichéd roles can reinforce outdated norms. Thus, media serves as both a mirror reflecting societal attitudes towards gender and a tool for shaping those perceptions.

Educational systems also play a significant role in molding gender expectations from an early age. Textbooks that highlight contributions from both men and women across various fields can foster a more balanced view among young learners. In contrast, curricula that overlook the achievements of women or minority groups contribute to maintaining skewed perceptions of gender capabilities.

Legislative frameworks reflect and influence societal norms regarding gender. Laws promoting equal rights and opportunities serve as benchmarks for societal progress towards gender equality. They not only provide mechanisms for addressing discrimination but also signal cultural shifts towards recognizing the importance of dismantling harmful stereotypes.

- Historical Context: Examining how past societal structures inform present-day gender expectations.

- Media Representation: Analyzing how media portrayals reinforce or challenge societal norms related to gender.

- Educational Systems: Exploring the role of education in shaping perceptions about gender from an early age.

- Legislative Frameworks: Assessing how laws reflect cultural attitudes towards gender equality.

In conclusion, society and culture are dynamic forces that continuously shape our understanding of gender roles. By examining these influences across different domains—historical context, media representation, educational systems, and legislative frameworks—we gain insights into how deeply entrenched beliefs about gender can be challenged and transformed for a more equitable future.

2

Cognitive Abilities and Preferences

2.1 Verbal and Mathematical Skills Across Genders

The exploration of verbal and mathematical skills across genders not only sheds light on cognitive differences but also provides insights into how these abilities influence professional choices, academic achievements, and interpersonal relationships. This nuanced understanding helps in debunking stereotypes and fostering a more inclusive environment where individual strengths are recognized beyond gender-based expectations.

Research indicates that on average, women tend to excel in verbal tasks, which include reading comprehension, writing ability, and language fluency. This proficiency can be attributed to both neurological and social factors. For instance, studies suggest that areas of the brain associated with language and fine motor skills may develop more rapidly in girls during childhood. Socially, girls are often encouraged from a young age to engage in activities that promote verbal expression, such as storytelling or playing with toys that involve complex narratives.

Conversely, men often show a predilection for mathematical and spatial reasoning tasks. This includes problem-solving in abstract spaces, mental rotation of objects, and higher performance in mathematics testing. The reasons behind these tendencies are multifaceted, involving evolutionary theories that link spatial skills to navigation and hunting roles historically attributed to men. Educational practices also play a significant role; boys are frequently encouraged to pursue activities like sports or video games that enhance spatial awareness.

- Neurological development differences: Brain imaging studies have shown variations in areas responsible for language processing between genders.

- Socialization patterns: Cultural expectations influence the types of play children engage in, potentially reinforcing certain cognitive skills over others.

- Educational influences: Gender biases in education can lead teachers to unconsciously encourage students towards subjects traditionally associated with their gender.

This discussion is not meant to pigeonhole individuals based on gender but rather to highlight trends that have been observed across large groups. It's crucial to recognize the variability within each gender; not all women will naturally excel at verbal tasks nor will all men inherently outperform in mathematical areas. Understanding these general tendencies allows for a more tailored approach in education and career counseling, ensuring individuals can leverage their strengths regardless of societal expectations.

In conclusion, while there are observable differences in verbal and mathematical skills across genders due to a combination of biological predispositions and social conditioning, it's important to foster environments where all individuals feel empowered to pursue their interests and develop their talents fully. By doing so, we move closer towards breaking down stereotypes and building a society that values diversity in cognitive abilities.

2.2 Emotional Intelligence and Spatial Reasoning: A Gendered Overview

The exploration of emotional intelligence and spatial reasoning from a gender perspective offers intriguing insights into cognitive abilities that significantly influence life outcomes, including career success, social relationships, and personal well-being. This section delves into the nuanced interplay between these cognitive domains and gender, expanding upon the foundational understanding established in the previous discussion on verbal and mathematical skills.

Emotional intelligence (EI), broadly defined as the ability to perceive, use, understand, manage, and regulate emotions effectively in oneself and others, has been observed to exhibit gender differences in various studies. Women are often reported to have higher EI than men, excelling particularly in empathy and interpersonal relationships. This difference is attributed to both biological predispositions and socialization patterns. For instance, neuroscientific research suggests that areas of the brain involved in emotion processing may differ between genders, potentially influencing emotional sensitivity and empathy levels. Socially, girls are frequently encouraged to express their feelings and develop strong communication skills from a young age—factors that contribute to enhanced emotional intelligence.

In contrast, spatial reasoning—the capacity to comprehend, reason about, and manipulate objects in three-dimensional space—shows a different pattern of gender disparity. Studies consistently demonstrate that men tend to outperform women on tasks requiring spatial visualization, such as mental rotation or navigation. This advantage is linked to evolutionary theories proposing that male-dominated hunter-gatherer roles necessitated superior spatial navigation skills. Additionally, societal influences play a significant role; boys are more likely encouraged to engage in activities like playing with building blocks or video games that enhance spatial skills.

- Biological underpinnings: Research indicates hormonal influences on brain development may contribute to observed differences in EI and spatial reasoning abilities across genders.

- Socialization practices: The types of play children are encouraged to participate in can reinforce certain cognitive strengths related to emotional understanding or spatial awareness.

- Educational implications: Recognizing these cognitive tendencies can inform teaching strategies that foster a more inclusive learning environment by supporting areas where students may face challenges while leveraging their natural strengths.

This gendered overview of emotional intelligence and spatial reasoning underscores the importance of considering both innate predispositions and environmental factors when examining cognitive abilities. It highlights the complexity of human cognition—a tapestry woven from threads of biological development, cultural expectations, personal experiences, and educational opportunities. By acknowledging these differences without succumbing to stereotypes or deterministic views on ability based on gender alone we can pave the way for more personalized approaches in education therapy career guidance ultimately enriching our collective human experience through diversity thought perspective emotion.

2.3 Motor Skills and Problem-Solving Strategies

The interconnection between motor skills and problem-solving strategies is a fascinating area of cognitive science that sheds light on how physical actions and cognitive processes are intertwined. This section explores the intricate relationship between these two domains, offering insights into how they influence each other and contribute to effective problem-solving in both everyday tasks and complex situations.

Motor skills, encompassing both fine and gross motor abilities, play a crucial role in executing tasks that require physical interaction with the environment. Fine motor skills involve small movements such as writing or manipulating small objects, while gross motor skills cover larger movements like walking or jumping. These physical abilities are not only essential for performing tasks but also significantly impact an individual's ability to engage with problem-solving activities.

Problem-solving strategies, on the other hand, are cognitive processes used to identify solutions to challenges or obstacles. These strategies can range from analytical thinking and logical reasoning to creative ideation and hypothesis testing. The effectiveness of these cognitive approaches can be greatly influenced by one's motor skills. For instance, the development of fine motor skills has been linked to improved cognitive functions such as attention and memory, which are critical components of successful problem-solving.

- Physical manipulation of objects often leads to enhanced spatial reasoning, allowing individuals to better visualize potential solutions.

- Engagement in activities that require coordination and movement can stimulate neural pathways associated with planning and strategy formulation.

- The act of writing or drawing during the problem-solving process can facilitate clearer thinking and idea organization.

This synergy between motor skills and cognitive strategies highlights the importance of incorporating physical activity into learning environments. Educational approaches that integrate movement with intellectual tasks—such as using manipulatives in mathematics or conducting experiments in science—can enhance understanding and retention of complex concepts. Moreover, recognizing the value of motor skill development in relation to cognitive abilities underscores the need for holistic educational practices that nurture both physical and mental growth.

In conclusion, the dynamic interplay between motor skills and problem-solving strategies illustrates a comprehensive view of human cognition that transcends traditional boundaries separating physical action from mental processes. By fostering both sets of skills simultaneously, individuals can enhance their capacity for innovative thinking, adaptability, and effective problem resolution in diverse aspects of life.

3

Evolutionary Adaptations and Modern Implications

3.1 Division of Labor in Ancient Societies

The division of labor in ancient societies was not merely a matter of assigning tasks but a complex system that reflected the social, economic, and environmental realities of the time. This system played a crucial role in the survival and development of these societies, allowing them to optimize resources, enhance productivity, and establish social hierarchies. The underlying principles of this division were deeply intertwined with the physical and intellectual differences observed between genders, which were then amplified by evolutionary pressures.

In hunter-gatherer communities, for instance, men typically took on roles that required brute strength and spatial awareness such as hunting and defending territory. Women, on the other hand, often engaged in gathering edible plants, preparing food, and caring for children. These roles exploited the natural strengths of each gender to ensure the group's survival. However, it's important to note that this division was not rigid; survival often necessitated flexibility and cooperation beyond strict gender lines.

Agricultural advancements led to more settled forms of society where the division of labor became more complex and specialized. Tasks were increasingly divided not just by gender but by skill sets, leading to the emergence of various professions. This specialization allowed societies to develop surplus goods which could be traded, laying the foundations for economic systems.

- Gender-based roles were influenced by physical attributes but were also shaped by societal needs.

- The transition from nomadic to settled life allowed for greater specialization in tasks.

- Specialization led to increased efficiency and the development of trade networks.

This early division of labor has left a lasting impact on modern societies. While today's world offers much more flexibility in terms of gender roles and employment opportunities, many contemporary divisions can trace their roots back to these ancient practices. Understanding this evolution helps us appreciate how far we have come in terms of equality and specialization while recognizing areas where traditional divisions persist or need reevaluation.

3.2 The Transition from Survival to Social Bonds in Human Evolution

The transition from survival strategies to the formation of complex social bonds marks a pivotal chapter in human evolution. This shift not only reflects changes in environmental and societal structures but also underscores the adaptive nature of humans in seeking not just survival, but also a thriving community. The importance of this transition lies in its profound impact on the development of social structures, cultures, and even cognitive abilities among early humans.

Initially, survival was predominantly about securing food, shelter, and protection against predators. Early humans lived in small groups or bands where cooperation was essential for hunting and gathering. However, as these groups became more successful at securing resources, the dynamics began to shift towards more permanent settlements. This change laid the groundwork for the development of social bonds that went beyond immediate family units to include larger community networks.

The establishment of these broader social bonds was facilitated by several key developments. The advent of language played a crucial role by enabling more sophisticated communication and collaboration among group members. Language allowed for the sharing of knowledge across generations, contributing to cultural evolution and the strengthening of social ties through shared beliefs and practices.

Agriculture was another significant milestone that influenced social bonding. As communities settled and began cultivating land, they became more stationary, leading to increased population density and necessitating more complex social structures for managing resources, labor division, and conflict resolution. These societies developed rituals, traditions, and norms that further solidified group cohesion and identity.

- Language facilitated complex communication and cultural transmission.
- Agriculture led to settled communities with denser populations.
- Rituals and traditions strengthened group cohesion.

This evolutionary journey from survival-focused bands to complex societies with intricate social bonds illustrates how human adaptation has been driven not only by biological needs but also by an inherent drive towards creating meaningful connections with others. Understanding this transition helps us appreciate the deep-rooted social nature of humans which continues to influence modern societal structures and interpersonal relationships.

3.3 Modern Family Dynamics and the Shift in Marriage Patterns

The evolution from survival-centric bands to complex social structures has not only shaped human societies historically but continues to influence contemporary family dynamics and marriage patterns. This section delves into the significant transformations in how modern families are formed, operate, and perceive the institution of marriage, reflecting broader societal changes and individual aspirations.

One of the most notable shifts is the increasing age at which individuals choose to marry. Economic factors, educational pursuits, and career advancements are often cited as reasons for this delay. This trend towards later marriages has implications for fertility rates and the structure of family units, with many opting to have fewer children or none at all. Additionally, there's a growing acceptance and prevalence of non-traditional family structures, including single-parent households, cohabiting couples without formal marriage bonds, and same-sex partnerships.

Technological advancements have also played a pivotal role in shaping modern relationships. Online dating platforms have transformed how people meet potential partners, broadening social networks beyond traditional community and cultural boundaries. This democratization of partner selection reflects a shift towards more individualistic values in mate choice, contrasting sharply with historical practices of arranged marriages that prioritized familial alliances over personal compatibility.

- Increased age at first marriage due to economic and personal aspirations.
- Rise in non-traditional family structures reflecting diverse societal acceptance.
- Impact of technology on partner selection and relationship formation.

The implications of these shifts are profound, affecting not just the immediate family unit but also wider societal norms around gender roles, parenting styles, and intergenerational support systems. For instance, as women increasingly participate in higher education and the workforce, traditional gender roles within marriages face reevaluation. Couples now navigate dual-career challenges while balancing domestic responsibilities in ways that diverge significantly from previous generations.

In conclusion, modern family dynamics and marriage patterns are characterized by diversity, choice, and adaptability. These changes reflect broader evolutionary trends towards social complexity but are uniquely shaped by contemporary cultural forces, technological innovations, and shifting individual priorities. Understanding these dynamics offers insights into the evolving nature of human relationships in response to changing environmental pressures and opportunities.

4

Navigating Relationships in the Contemporary World

4.1 The Importance of Negotiation and Agreement in Partnerships

In the contemporary world, where traditional roles within partnerships are increasingly fluid and subject to personal choice rather than societal expectation, the importance of negotiation and agreement cannot be overstated. This shift from predefined roles towards a more egalitarian model necessitates a deeper understanding and application of negotiation skills to ensure harmony and mutual satisfaction in relationships.

Negotiation and agreement serve as the bedrock for successful partnerships by fostering an environment where both parties feel heard, valued, and respected. This process allows individuals to express their needs, desires, and expectations openly without fear of judgment or reprisal. In doing so, it not only bridges intellectual differences but also accommodates varying emotional needs and preferences that may exist between partners.

The evolution from traditional gender roles towards a more balanced partnership underscores the need for negotiation. Historically, roles were often assigned based on gender, with little room for deviation or discussion. However, as society progresses towards valuing individual strengths and competencies over traditional gender assignments, couples must engage in ongoing dialogue to determine who is best suited for various responsibilities within the relationship.

- Effective communication strategies are essential for successful negotiation; this includes active listening, empathy, and the ability to articulate one's own needs clearly.

- Conflict resolution skills play a crucial role in reaching agreements that satisfy both parties. Understanding how to compromise without feeling compromised is key.

- Setting clear boundaries and expectations from the outset can prevent misunderstandings and resentment later on.

Negotiation is not just about resolving conflicts or delegating tasks; it's about building a foundation of trust and respect that strengthens the partnership over time. By embracing negotiation as a tool for mutual growth rather than a hurdle to overcome, couples can create dynamic relationships that adapt to life's changes while maintaining a core of stability and support.

In conclusion, as we navigate relationships in today's complex social landscape, the ability to negotiate effectively stands out as an indispensable skill. It enables partners to celebrate their differences while working together towards common goals—ultimately enriching their partnership with depth, understanding, and enduring affection.

4.2 Complementary Skills and Interests Within Relationships

The dynamic of complementary skills and interests plays a pivotal role in the fabric of contemporary relationships, acting as a cornerstone for mutual growth and enrichment. This concept extends beyond the traditional division of labor to encompass a broader spectrum of personal and professional development opportunities within partnerships. By leveraging individual strengths, couples can create a synergistic relationship that not only fosters personal fulfillment but also strengthens their bond.

In today's world, where individuality and personal growth are highly valued, the ability to support and complement each other's skills and interests is invaluable. This approach encourages partners to explore new territories together or individually, knowing they have a supportive base to return to. It's about recognizing that one partner's strength can compensate for the other's weakness, thereby creating a balanced and resilient union.

- Emotional intelligence plays a significant role in identifying and nurturing complementary skills within relationships. It allows partners to communicate effectively, recognize each other's needs, and provide support where it's most needed.

- Shared interests serve as common ground for couples, offering opportunities for bonding and experiencing joy together. Meanwhile, respecting individual interests encourages independence and self-expression—key components of a healthy relationship.

- Diverse skill sets enable couples to tackle life's challenges more efficiently. When one partner excels in financial management while the other shines in creative problem-solving, they cover more ground together than they would individually.

This integration of complementary skills and interests requires ongoing communication and adjustment as individuals evolve over time. What begins as an alignment of professional skills might blossom into shared hobbies or vice versa. The beauty lies in the journey of discovery—learning about each other's evolving passions and capabilities while navigating life's complexities together.

In conclusion, embracing complementary skills and interests within relationships is not merely about enhancing compatibility; it's about actively contributing to each other's happiness and success. As partners learn from one another, they not only enrich their relationship but also pave the way for a fulfilling life journey together.

4.3 Overcoming Traditional Gender Roles in Modern Partnerships

The evolution of societal norms has significantly impacted the dynamics within modern partnerships, challenging traditional gender roles and fostering a more egalitarian approach to relationship building. This shift is not just about redistributing household chores but also about redefining emotional labor, decision-making processes, and professional support between partners. Overcoming these traditional roles requires conscious effort, open communication, and a willingness to embrace change for the betterment of both individuals involved.

At the heart of this transformation is the recognition that adherence to rigid gender roles can limit personal growth and mutual satisfaction within a partnership. For instance, the expectation that men should always be the primary breadwinners or that women should handle all domestic responsibilities is increasingly seen as outdated. Instead, modern couples are finding value in sharing these roles or alternating them based on current life circumstances, such as career demands or personal preferences.

- Communication is key to navigating this shift; partners must feel comfortable discussing their expectations, desires, and concerns without fear of judgment.

- Flexibility allows couples to adapt their roles as needed rather than being confined by societal norms or stereotypes.

- Supporting each other's careers and personal goals can strengthen the relationship by demonstrating mutual respect and admiration for each other's ambitions.

This new paradigm encourages partners to view their relationship as a partnership of equals, where both individuals contribute according to their strengths and preferences rather than predetermined roles. It acknowledges that every couple is unique and what works for one may not work for another. Therefore, overcoming traditional gender roles is less about adhering to a specific formula and more about creating a bespoke arrangement that aligns with the values and aspirations of both partners.

In conclusion, while overcoming traditional gender roles presents its challenges, it also offers an opportunity for deeper connection and understanding between partners. By fostering an environment of equality, respect, and support, modern partnerships can thrive beyond conventional constraints—leading to richer, more fulfilling relationships.

5

Redefining Roles in the Twenty-First Century

5.1 The Disappearance of Traditional Gender Expectations

The evolution of societal norms has led to a significant shift in the roles traditionally expected of men and women, particularly in the context of family and work dynamics. This transformation is rooted in both the changing economic landscape and the progressive recognition of gender equality. As we delve into this topic, it's essential to understand how these shifts contribute to redefining roles in the twenty-first century, moving away from rigid gender expectations towards a more fluid understanding of capabilities and preferences.

Historically, gender roles were clearly defined, with men typically seen as breadwinners and women as homemakers. These roles were not only socially enforced but were also legally codified, limiting opportunities for women in particular. However, the latter half of the twentieth century saw a dramatic change in this paradigm due to several factors including increased female participation in the workforce, higher education levels among women, and a growing awareness of gender rights.

The disappearance of traditional gender expectations can be attributed to several key developments:

This evolution towards egalitarian relationships reflects broader societal changes where individual preferences and competencies are valued over traditional norms. Couples now often negotiate roles based on personal strengths, interests, and economic considerations rather than defaulting to pre-determined gender-based responsibilities. This shift not only allows for greater flexibility within relationships but also challenges stereotypes that limit what individuals can achieve based on their gender.

- **Economic Necessity:** The economic demands of modern living require most families to have dual incomes. This necessity has pushed both men and women into the workforce, making it less feasible for one partner to remain solely responsible for home management.

- **Educational Attainment:** Women now surpass men in educational attainment in many parts of the world. This shift has opened up new opportunities for women while also challenging traditional notions about gender-specific roles in society.

- **Societal Acceptance:** There's been a significant move towards accepting diverse family structures and rejecting stereotypes that dictate what men and women can or cannot do. This acceptance promotes an environment where individuals feel free to pursue careers and lifestyles irrespective of their gender.

- **Technological Advancements:** Technology has simplified tasks that were once physically demanding or time-consuming, reducing the need for traditional divisions of labor based on physical strength or availability at home.

In conclusion, the disappearance of traditional gender expectations marks a significant step towards achieving true equality between men and women. By recognizing that abilities are not inherently tied to one's sex, society opens up a realm of possibilities where individuals can excel based on their talents and passions rather than being constrained by outdated norms.

5.2 Homemaking and Career: Finding Balance Beyond Gender

The quest for balance between homemaking and career pursuits transcends traditional gender roles, reflecting a modern society's aspirations for equality and personal fulfillment. This evolution mirrors the broader societal shift towards recognizing individual capabilities over gender-prescribed roles, as detailed in the disappearance of traditional gender expectations. The dual pursuit of career ambitions alongside homemaking responsibilities presents both challenges and opportunities for individuals, irrespective of their gender.

In this context, finding balance involves navigating economic realities, personal aspirations, and societal expectations to forge a path that accommodates both professional growth and a fulfilling home life. The increasing participation of both men and women in the workforce has necessitated a more equitable distribution of domestic responsibilities. This shift is not merely economic but deeply rooted in changing perceptions about what individuals can achieve regardless of their gender.

Technological advancements have played a pivotal role in facilitating this balance by streamlining household tasks and enabling flexible work arrangements. Remote work options, for instance, allow individuals to manage their professional responsibilities without compromising on their presence at home. Similarly, modern appliances and digital tools have reduced the time and physical effort required for domestic chores, making it easier for all members of a household to contribute to homemaking tasks.

The journey towards balancing homemaking with career aspirations is highly individualized, shaped by factors such as career goals, family dynamics, personal values, and societal pressures. Couples increasingly engage in open dialogues to distribute tasks equitably based on workload capacities rather than defaulting to traditional allocations based on gender. This negotiation process is crucial in fostering supportive relationships that accommodate the ambitions and well-being of all members.

- **Economic Imperatives:** The necessity for dual incomes in many households has blurred traditional distinctions between breadwinners and homemakers, pushing couples to negotiate shared responsibilities based on practical considerations rather than societal norms.

- **Educational Achievements:** With women achieving higher levels of education and entering professions historically dominated by men, there's been a recalibration of expectations around who pursues careers versus who tends to home duties.

- **Societal Shifts:** A growing acceptance of diverse family structures encourages a more fluid approach to dividing labor at home, allowing individuals to tailor their roles according to personal strengths and preferences rather than rigid gender stereotypes.

- **Technological Ease:** The simplification of household management through technology empowers individuals to efficiently juggle career demands with domestic responsibilities.

In conclusion, transcending traditional gender roles to find harmony between career ambitions and homemaking is an evolving narrative in the twenty-first century. It reflects broader changes towards egalitarianism within societies valuing diversity, flexibility, and mutual respect over outdated norms. By focusing on abilities rather than predetermined roles, individuals can craft fulfilling lives that honor both their professional aspirations and the importance of a nurturing home environment.

5.3 Seeking Completeness in Partnerships Regardless of Gender

In the evolving landscape of modern relationships, the pursuit of completeness within partnerships, irrespective of gender, marks a significant departure from traditional paradigms. This shift is not merely about redistributing domestic chores or sharing financial burdens but encompasses a deeper quest for emotional fulfillment, mutual respect, and shared life goals. As society progresses towards a more inclusive understanding of gender roles, individuals are increasingly looking beyond conventional expectations to form partnerships that are truly symbiotic.

The essence of seeking completeness lies in recognizing and valuing each partner's contributions, strengths, and aspirations without the constraints imposed by gender stereotypes. This approach fosters an environment where both individuals can thrive personally and professionally, supporting each other's ambitions while nurturing a shared vision for their future together. It challenges the outdated notion that one's biological sex predetermines their role within a relationship or family structure.

- **Emotional Intelligence:** A key component in these partnerships is the emphasis on emotional intelligence—understanding and managing one's own emotions as well as empathizing with one's partner. This skill set enables couples to navigate conflicts more effectively, share responsibilities more equitably, and support each other's growth.

- **Diverse Family Models:** The acceptance and celebration of diverse family structures play a crucial role in redefining partnership roles. By witnessing and acknowledging various successful models—from single-parent families to same-sex couples raising children—society broadens its perspective on what it means to be a supportive partner or parent.

- **Professional Flexibility:** With the rise of remote work and flexible schedules, couples have more leeway to design their professional lives in a way that complements their personal commitments. This flexibility is instrumental in allowing both partners to pursue career excellence without sacrificing their involvement at home.

This holistic approach to partnership transcends traditional gender roles and focuses on creating balanced relationships where both individuals feel valued and fulfilled. By prioritizing communication, equality, and respect, couples can build strong foundations that support both partners' desires for personal achievement and happiness within the relationship. In doing so, they contribute to a broader societal shift towards inclusivity and mutual support that enriches communities as a whole.

In conclusion, seeking completeness in partnerships regardless of gender represents an enlightened path forward in human relationships. It embodies the principles of equality, diversity, and personal fulfillment that are increasingly recognized as essential for thriving societies. As we continue to challenge old norms and embrace new possibilities, these partnerships will undoubtedly play a pivotal role in shaping a more equitable world.

6

Gender Equality in Education and Career Opportunities

6.1 The Gender Gap in STEM Fields

The gender gap in Science, Technology, Engineering, and Mathematics (STEM) fields is a significant issue that reflects broader societal inequalities. This disparity not only limits the diversity of perspectives in these crucial areas but also restricts women's access to some of the most lucrative and influential careers. Understanding the roots and ramifications of this gap is essential for devising effective strategies to close it.

Historically, STEM fields have been male-dominated, with cultural and educational systems often discouraging women from pursuing these paths. Stereotypes suggesting that men are more naturally suited to math and science further exacerbate this imbalance. However, research shows that the performance gap in math between boys and girls in school is minimal, suggesting that differences in achievement are not due to innate ability.

One major factor contributing to the gender gap in STEM is the lack of female role models. Women who might have pursued careers in these fields often face isolation and a lack of mentorship, leading many to abandon these paths. Additionally, workplace environments in STEM industries can be unwelcoming or even hostile to women, characterized by gender bias and discrimination.

In conclusion, closing the gender gap in STEM requires a multifaceted approach that addresses cultural stereotypes, educational barriers, workplace environments, and the need for mentorship and role models. By tackling these issues head-on, society can unlock a wealth of untapped potential and move towards true equality both within STEM fields and beyond.

- Lack of Female Role Models: The scarcity of women in senior positions within STEM fields discourages younger generations from pursuing similar careers.

- Educational Barriers: Gender biases in education can steer girls away from math and science as early as primary school.

- Cultural Stereotypes: Persistent stereotypes about gender roles can dissuade girls from developing an interest in STEM subjects.

- Workplace Environment: Discrimination and a lack of support within STEM workplaces can deter women from remaining in these fields long-term.

To bridge this gap, concerted efforts are needed at multiple levels. Initiatives aimed at encouraging girls' participation in STEM from an early age are crucial. This includes creating more inclusive educational materials, providing mentorship programs that connect young women with female leaders in STEM, and fostering a culture that challenges stereotypes rather than perpetuating them. Moreover, addressing workplace cultures to make them more inclusive and supportive for women is essential for retaining talent and ensuring diverse perspectives contribute to innovation within these fields.

6.2 Overcoming Stereotypes and Bias in Education and Career Choices

The journey to overcoming stereotypes and bias in education and career choices is pivotal for achieving gender equality. This challenge is deeply rooted in societal norms that have historically dictated the roles deemed appropriate for men and women. The impact of these stereotypes extends beyond personal choices, influencing the broader landscape of professional fields and contributing to the persistent gender gaps observed in various sectors, notably STEM (Science, Technology, Engineering, Mathematics).

Addressing these biases requires a multifaceted approach that begins with early education. Schools play a crucial role in either perpetuating or dismantling gender stereotypes. By integrating curriculum materials that showcase diverse role models and emphasize the achievements of women in traditionally male-dominated fields, educators can begin to reshape perceptions from a young age. Furthermore, creating classroom environments that encourage all students equally to explore their interests in subjects like math and science is essential.

Beyond educational settings, media representation also significantly influences career aspirations. The portrayal of female professionals in STEM careers on television shows, movies, and online platforms can inspire young girls to pursue similar paths. Efforts to increase visibility of women excelling in these areas help normalize the presence of women in high-level scientific roles, challenging the stereotype that these careers are not suited for them.

- Early Educational Interventions: Implementing programs that expose students to STEM fields through hands-on activities and real-world applications can spark interest among girls at a young age.

- Mentorship Programs: Connecting young women with mentors in their field of interest provides guidance, support, and inspiration. These relationships can demystify the path to success in male-dominated industries.

- Inclusive Workplace Cultures: Companies must actively work towards creating environments that support diversity and inclusion. This includes implementing policies against discrimination, providing equal opportunities for advancement, and recognizing unconscious biases within hiring practices.

To dismantle long-standing stereotypes effectively requires concerted efforts across multiple domains—education systems must evolve; media representations need to be more inclusive; workplaces should foster diversity and equality; and policy interventions may be necessary to ensure equitable access to opportunities. By addressing these areas collectively, society can move closer towards eliminating gender bias in education and career choices, paving the way for a future where individuals are free to pursue their passions without constraint by outdated societal expectations.

6.3 Promoting Equal Opportunities for Women in Leadership Positions

The advancement of women into leadership positions is a critical aspect of achieving gender equality across various sectors. Despite progress in some areas, significant barriers remain that prevent women from accessing and thriving in these roles. This section delves into strategies and initiatives aimed at promoting equal opportunities for women in leadership, expanding on the foundational efforts to overcome stereotypes and biases outlined previously.

Creating pathways for women to ascend to leadership roles involves addressing both systemic barriers and cultural perceptions. One effective approach is the implementation of targeted leadership development programs. These programs are designed not only to equip women with the necessary skills but also to boost their confidence in their ability to lead. By focusing on mentorship, networking opportunities, and training in areas such as negotiation and strategic decision-making, these initiatives can play a pivotal role in preparing women for leadership.

- Leadership Development Programs: Tailored initiatives that provide training, mentorship, and networking opportunities specifically for aspiring female leaders.

- Sponsorship: Encouraging senior leaders to actively sponsor high-potential women by advocating for their advancement and exposing them to strategic opportunities.

- Flexible Work Arrangements: Implementing policies that support work-life balance, enabling women to pursue leadership roles without sacrificing personal or family commitments.

Beyond individual development, organizational culture plays a significant role in either facilitating or hindering the progression of women into leadership positions. Cultivating an inclusive culture that values diversity at all levels—including gender diversity—is essential. This includes critically examining recruitment, promotion practices, and performance evaluation criteria to identify and eliminate biases that may disadvantage women candidates. Additionally, transparency around career progression paths and criteria for advancement can demystify the process for aspiring female leaders.

To complement internal efforts, policy interventions at the national or industry level can also have a profound impact. Legislation mandating gender diversity on corporate boards or within certain sectors can accelerate change by setting clear targets and accountability mechanisms. Moreover, public campaigns highlighting successful female leaders across various fields serve not only as inspiration but also help challenge outdated stereotypes about what effective leadership looks like.

In conclusion, promoting equal opportunities for women in leadership positions requires a comprehensive approach that addresses both structural barriers and cultural norms. By combining targeted development programs with organizational changes and supportive policies, it is possible to create environments where women's leadership potential can be fully realized.

The book "Accept Our Differences" delves into the nuanced intellectual differences between men and women, attributing these variances to evolutionary processes shaped by ancient societal roles. It highlights how, on average, women tend to excel in verbal tasks and possess higher emotional skills, while men are generally better at math-based activities and spatial reasoning. The text explores how these differences were essential for survival in early human societies, where task division between genders was a necessity for managing daily life challenges.

Despite the evolution of society towards more individualistic lifestyles where single-headed families are common and marriage is not a survival necessity, the book argues that the desire for companionship remains strong. It emphasizes the importance of negotiation and agreement in relationships, suggesting that partners should complement each other's skills and interests to maintain harmony. The traditional gender roles have evolved, making it less about conforming to expected societal norms and more about finding a partner who completes you as an individual.

"Accept Our Differences" offers insightful perspectives on how understanding and embracing the inherent intellectual differences between genders can lead to more fulfilling relationships. It encourages readers to appreciate these distinctions not as barriers but as opportunities for growth and mutual support within partnerships. By doing so, it presents a modern approach to navigating gender dynamics that honors our evolutionary past while promoting equality and cooperation in contemporary society.

* 9 7 9 8 3 2 5 6 6 6 0 7 0 *